Myelodysplastic Syndrome:
Fast Focus Study Guide

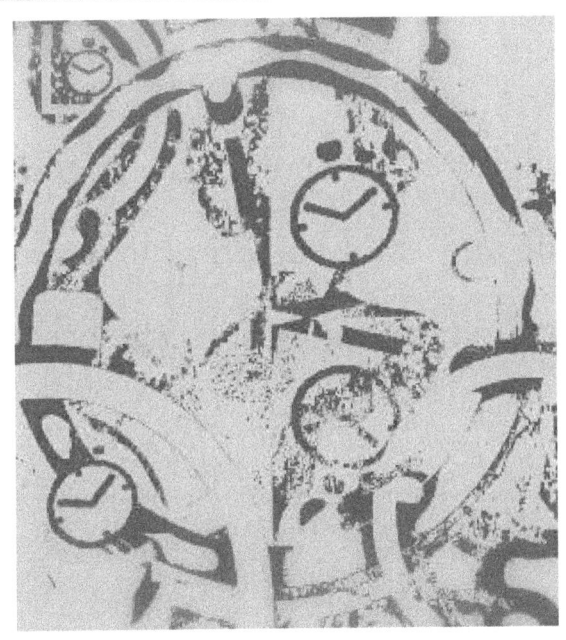

Acknowledgements

I dedicate this book to my beautiful wife and children, who I love more than all the water in all the oceans and all the seas.

CONTENTS

- This book is written for a medical student, resident, fellow, or attending physician who wants to better understand Myelodysplastic syndromes.

- This book is composed of easy to read facts that every doctor likely knows.

- Put this book in your bathroom or on your coffee table.

- This is the perfect book for someone who is preparing for boards.

- This Fast Focus Study Guide will provide you with a practical review of the key information you need to know.

- Buy this book now if you want this quick and concise information

Myelodysplastic syndromes (MDS) are a group of several related disorders characterized by bone marrow dysplasia and dysfunction associated with peripheral blood anemia, thrombocytopenia and or leukopenia.

Anemia is the most common finding in patients with MDS. The peripheral blood smear can show macrocytosis of the red cells and hypogranular neutrophils. The neutrophils can also show Pelger -Huet nuclei and other abnormal nuclear patterns and rarely you can see circulating micro megakaryocytes.

The myelodysplastic disorders can evolve over time into acute leukemia. There are nine defined myelodysplastic syndromes.

Age is a very important risk factor for the development of MDS.

Smoking is associated with a three to five-fold
increase in occurrence of myelodysplastic
syndrome.

MDS is a is disease of the elderly. It is rare in people less than 50 years old. MDS presents most commonly with symptoms of anemia.

The bone marrow in patients with MDS is typically hyper cellular which points to ineffective hematopoiesis as the cause of low cell counts.

Approximately 50% of patients with myelodysplastic syndromes have RAS mutations.

Approximately 15% of patients with myelodysplastic syndrome will have a monoclonal gammopathy.

The following pages describe the different types of MDS.

Refractory anemia is characterized by isolated anemia with normal white blood cell and platelet counts. There are <5% blasts in the marrow. This disorder is one of the low risk MDS.

Refractory anemia with ring sideroblasts is similar to refractory anemia except that at least 15% of marrow red cell precursors are ring sideroblasts. This is the second low risk MDS.

Refractory anemia with excess blasts (RAEB) is characterized by disordered myelopoiesis, megakaryocytopoiesis and erythropoiesis. This is subcategorized into RAEB-1 and RAEB-2. RAEB-1 is characterized by 5% to 9% blasts in the bone marrow and less than 5% blasts in the blood. RAEB-2 is characterized by 10% to 19% blasts in the bone marrow. Both categories of RAEB are considered high risk MDS.

The blast count in MDS may vary from less than 5% in refractory anemia (RA) to more than 5% blasts in refractory anemia with excess blasts (RAEB). A blast-cell count greater than 20% in the bone marrow defines the condition as acute leukemia.

Refractory cytopenia with multilineage dysplasia is characterized by bicytopenia or pancytopenia. Dysplastic changes are present in 10% or more of the cells in two or more myeloid cell lines. There are less than 1% blasts in the blood and less than 5% blasts in the bone marrow. Auer rods are not present. Monocytes in the blood are less than 1×10^9.

Refractory cytopenia with multilineage dysplasia and ring sideroblasts (RCMD-RS) is a subcategory characterized by more than 15% of erythroid precursors in the bone marrow are ring sideroblasts.

Refractory cytopenia with unilineage dysplasia is characterized by a single cytopenia involving either erythrocytes, neutrophils, or platelets. In addition, dysplastic changes are present in 10% or more of the cells in two or more myeloid cell lines. There are less than 1% blasts in the blood and less than 5% blasts in the bone marrow. Auer rods are not present. Monocytes in the blood are less than 1 × 109.

Unclassifiable myelodysplastic syndrome lacks findings appropriate for classification as RA, RARS, RCMD, or RAEB. Blasts in the blood and bone marrow are not increased.

Myelodysplastic syndrome associated with an isolated Del (5q) chromosome abnormality is associated with an isolated Del (5q) cytogenetic abnormality. Blasts in both blood and bone marrow are less than 5%.

The 5q MDS syndrome has a female predominance and often presents with macrocytic anemia, thrombocytosis, preserved neutrophil count, increased number of hypo lobulated and micro megakaryocytes.

Therapy-related MDS is seen in patients who were previously treated with chemotherapy or radiation therapy for other cancers and in whom there is a clinical suspicion that the prior therapy caused the myeloid neoplasm. Associated chemotherapies include alkylating agents, topoisomerase inhibitors, and purine analogs.

Therapy related MDS have a 75% chance of progressing to acute leukemia. The delay from exposure to chemotherapy or radiation to the development of secondary MDS is typically 2 to 10 years.

Alkylating agents (like cyclophosphamide) are associated with deletions in chromosomes 5 and/or 7.

Topoisomerase II inhibitors (like etoposide) are associated with 11q23 abnormalities and have a shorter delay than alkylating agents from exposure to diagnosis of MDS.

Chronic myelomonocytic leukemia (CMML) is assigned to a group of overlap myelodysplastic/myeloproliferative neoplasms.

Although we have the two prognostic scoring systems (IPSS and IPSS-R), the marrow blast-cell count is the single most important factor in determining prognosis, with a higher blast count conferring a poorer prognosis.

We also know that abnormalities in chromosome 7 and a complex karyotype are prominent high risk features that predispose to evolution to AML.

The IPSS-R is a standardized scoring system that helps determine the prognosis at the time of initial diagnosis based on cytogenetics, cytopenias, and bone marrow blast percentage. The following page outlines the details of the IPSS-R.

Table. The International Prognostic Scoring System (IPSS-R) for myelodysplastic syndromes (MDS)

Factor	Value	IPSS-R score
Blasts in bone marrow	≤2%	0
	>2%-<5%	1
	5->10%	2
	>10%	3
Cell DNA changes (cytogenetics)	Very good	0
	Good	1
	Intermediate	2
	Poor	3
	Very poor	4
Hemoglobin	≥10 g/dL	0
	8-< g/dL	1
	<8 g/dL	1.5
Platelets	≥100x10^9/L	0
	50-<100x10^9/L	0.5
	<50x10^9/L	1
ANC	≥0.8x10^9/L	0
	<0.8x10^9/L	0.5

The IPSS-R scoring system is used only at the time of MDS diagnosis as it does not take into account the impact of transfusions on the prognosis of MDS patients.

Based on these and other prognostic factors, the IPSS-R stratifies patients into risk categories by score:
- *Very low (≤1.5)*
- *Low: (1.5-3)*
- *Intermediate (3-4.5)*
- *High: (4.5-6)*
- *Very high (>6)*

In addition to the IPSS and the IPSS-R, we also now understood that highly complex TP53 mutant patients have the poorest survival risk.

Deletion 11q is a cytogenetic abnormality
associated with a good prognosis.

5q-, 20q-, and normal cytogenetics are also associated with better prognosis in patients with myelodysplastic syndrome.

We talk quite a bit about abnormal cytogenetics, but approximately 50 % of MDS patients will have a normal cytogenetics. Normal cytogenetics are associated with a good prognosis.

Additional cytogenetics associated with poor outcome include del 20q, and -Y.

Patients with an IPSS score of 1 or less or an IPSS-R score of 4 or less are considered low risk MDS.

If a patient has low risk MDS and anemia with the Del (5q) the treatment should include Lenalidomide.

When Lenalidomide was used in patients with the 5q- gene abnormality, transfusion independence was achieved in 67% of patients. Approximately 45% of patients achieved a complete cytogenetic remission, and the duration of response with > 2 years.

If a patient has low risk MDS and anemia without the Del (5q) and the serum erythropoietin is >500 the treatment is unclear.

If a patient has low risk MDS and anemia without the Del (5q) and the serum erythropoietin is < 500 U/L the treatment should include ESA with or without G-CSF.

Patients who need less than 2 units of red blood cells per month and have a serum erythropoietin level less than 500 U/ L have a >70% probability of responding to erythropoietin plus G-CSF.

If a patient has low risk MDS with neutropenia and/or thrombocytopenia there is no standard of care. The patient can be treated with growth factors, decitabine, or Azacitidine.

Patients with an IPSS score of 2 or more or an IPSS-R score of 5 or more are considered to have high risk MDS.

Azacitidine and decitabine are 2 common treatments for high risk MDS. These chemotherapies inhibit DNA methyltransferase and results in DNA hypo methylation.

A randomized trial of decitabine versus observation showed no survival benefit, but delayed time to AML.

(Lubbert et al, JCO 30:1987-1997, 2011)

Azacitidine was studied in high risk MDS and compared to conventional care regimens. The median survival in the patients treated with Azacitidine was 24.4 months versus 15 months for supportive care. The two year survival was 50.8% for Azacitidine versus 26.2%.

Fenaux P, et al. Lancet Oncology 2009;10:223-232

When Lenalidomide was used in patients who did not have the 5q- gene abnormality, transfusion independence was achieved in 26% of patients. Approximately 9% of patients achieved a complete cytogenetic remission, and the duration of response was approximately 41 weeks.

If a patient has high risk MDS and they are a candidate for transplant then the treatment should proceed toward transplant.

If a patient has high risk MDS and they are
not a candidate for transplant then the
treatment should include Azacitidine or
decitabine.

When patients have neutropenia or thrombocytopenia without excess blasts in the marrow, it is possible that the pathophysiology could be T-cell mediated in patients with MDS that do not have excessive blasts. There is data using cyclosporine, anti thymocyte globulin and even alemtuzumab in this setting.

This concludes Myelodysplasia: Fast Focus Study Guide

Search Amazon Kindle books to find other study guides written by

JT Thomas, MD

Multiple Myeloma Study Guide

Differential Diagnosis Study Guide

Rheumatology Study Guide

www.ingramcontent.com/pod-product-compliance
Lightning Source LLC
Chambersburg PA
CBHW071003180526
45168CB00003B/1275